StayC Bee and the Power of Hope

by Stayc Sharrow

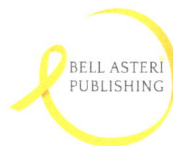

I0025394

BELL ASTERI
PUBLISHING

StayC Bee and the Power of Hope

Copyright ©2026 by Stayc Sharrow

Author: Stayc Sharrow
Illustrators: Destiny and Sam

Published by Bell Asteri Publishing & Enterprises, LLC
209 West 2nd Street #177
Fort Worth TX 76102
www.bellasteri.com

Published in the United States of America

ISBN: 978-1-957604-82-4

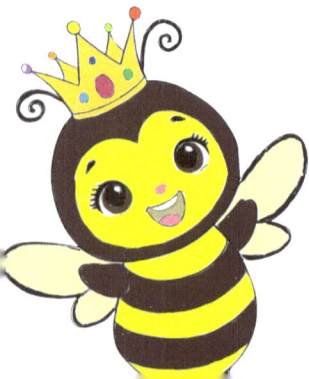

In loving memory of Elise and all those we've lost to cancer, and in honor of Michael and every brave thriver. With love to Ashlee and all the caregivers who bring hope each day. May I make you proud.

With deepest gratitude to the best support team: Scot, Ang, Gary, Mike, Debi, Jean, and Christen.

And to my incredible worker bees: Ale, Amanda M., Amanda K., Amy, Ana Sofia, Angie, Ashley, Diego, Gennesis, Justin, Malaya, and Mari. Thank you for your dedication and heart.

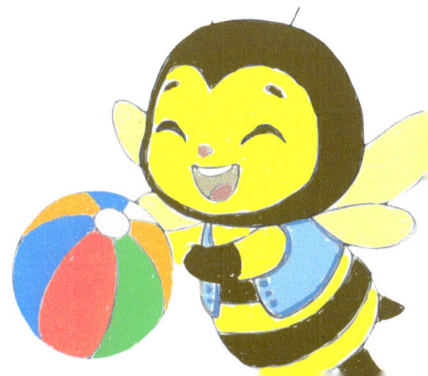

In a sunny garden by a sparkling river stood a happy, buzzing beehive. The hive was full of love and laughter, ruled by the kind and cheerful Queen Bee who had a brave, beautiful daughter named StayC.

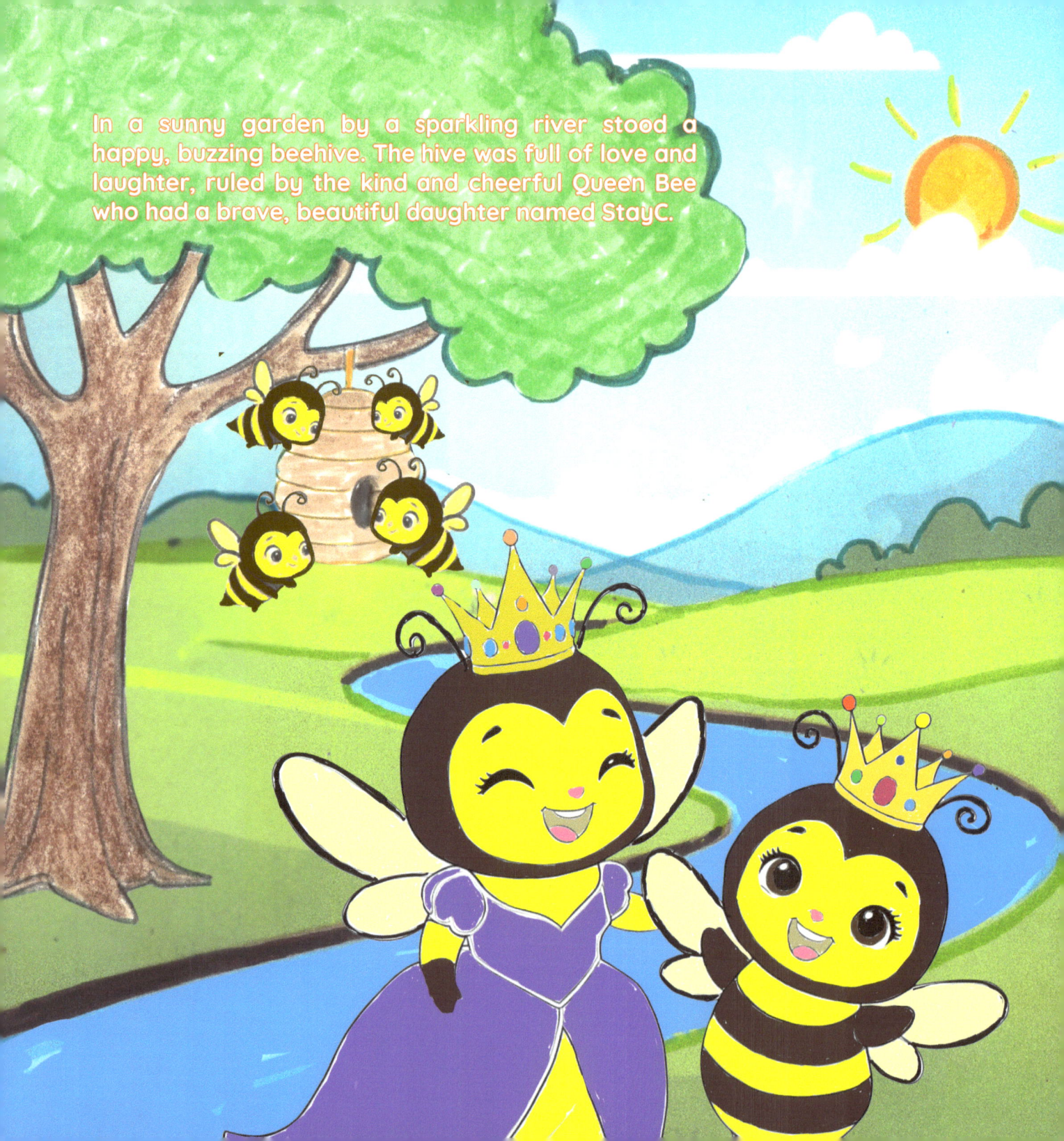

StayC Bee's best friend was Sir Scot, the happiest, funniest bee in the hive. They played together every day, told funny stories, and made sure all the bees in the hive felt loved.

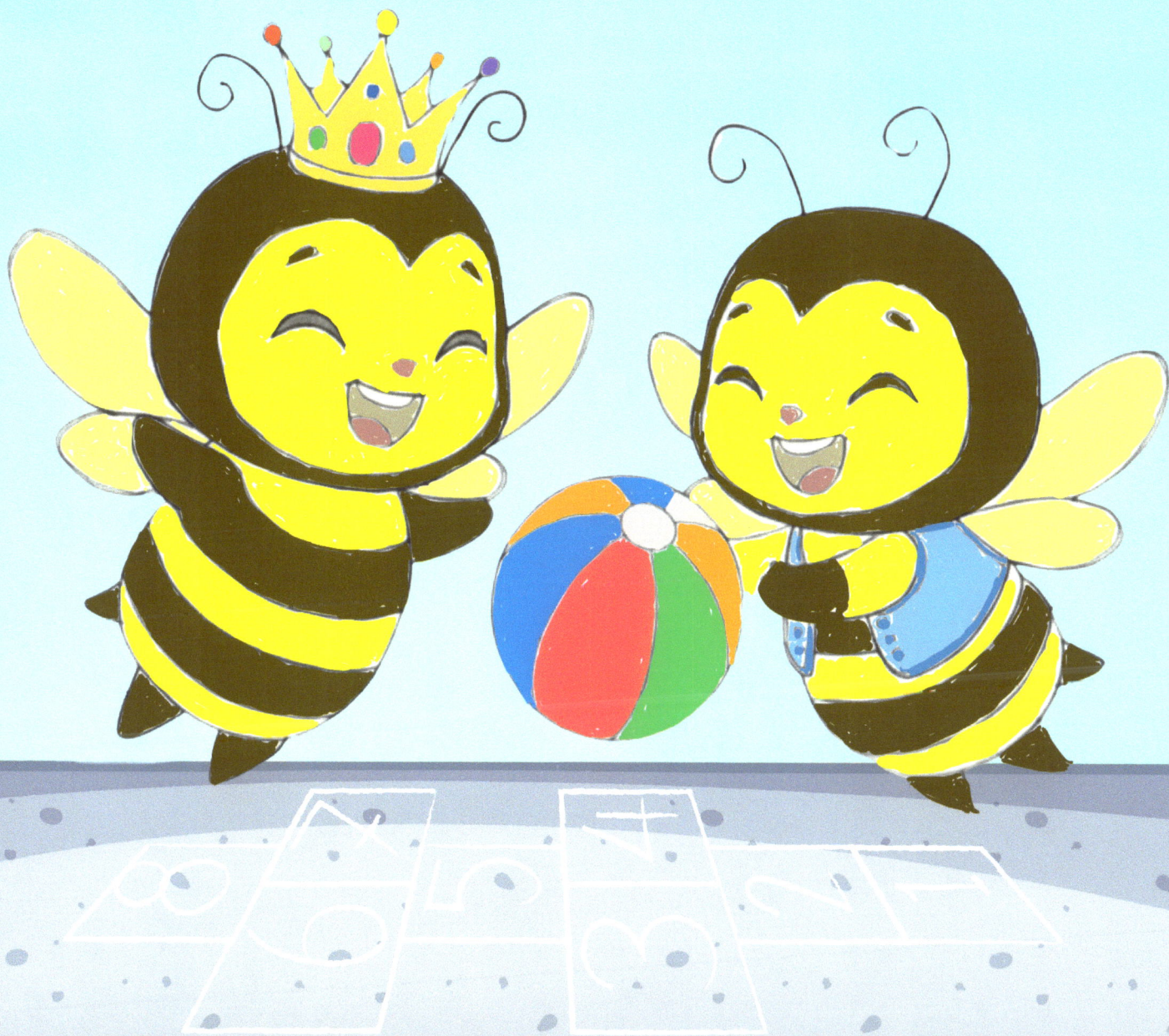

Every day, StayC Bee flew through the garden her mom had planted for her, checking on her flowers and waving to her friends. Her golden crown shimmered in the sunlight, and her wings sparkled like stars.

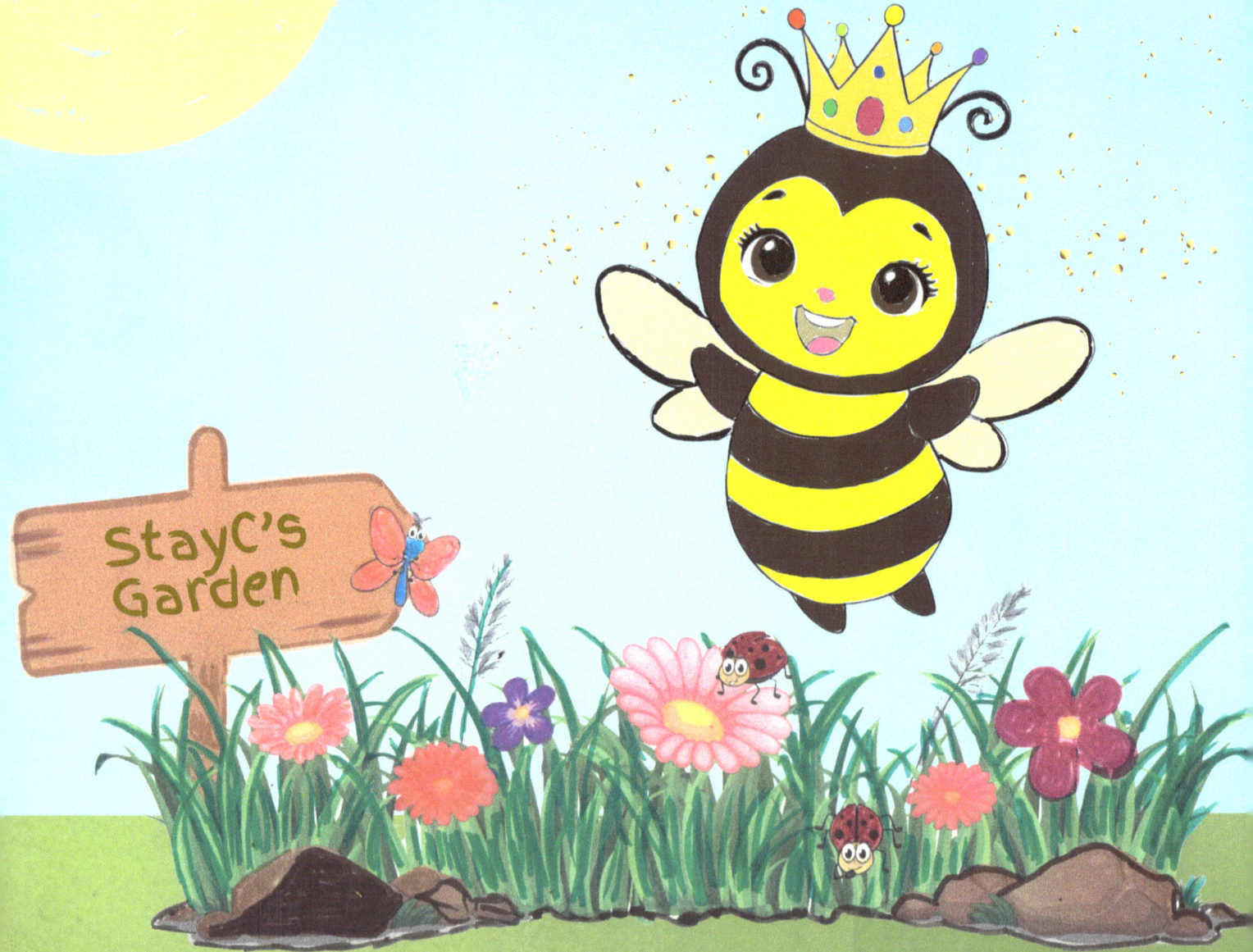

StayC's Garden

But one day, something unexpected happened. As StayC Bee was flying near her favorite flower, she suddenly felt dizzy and fell to the ground. Queen Bee, Sir Scot, and the other bees rushed over to see what was wrong.

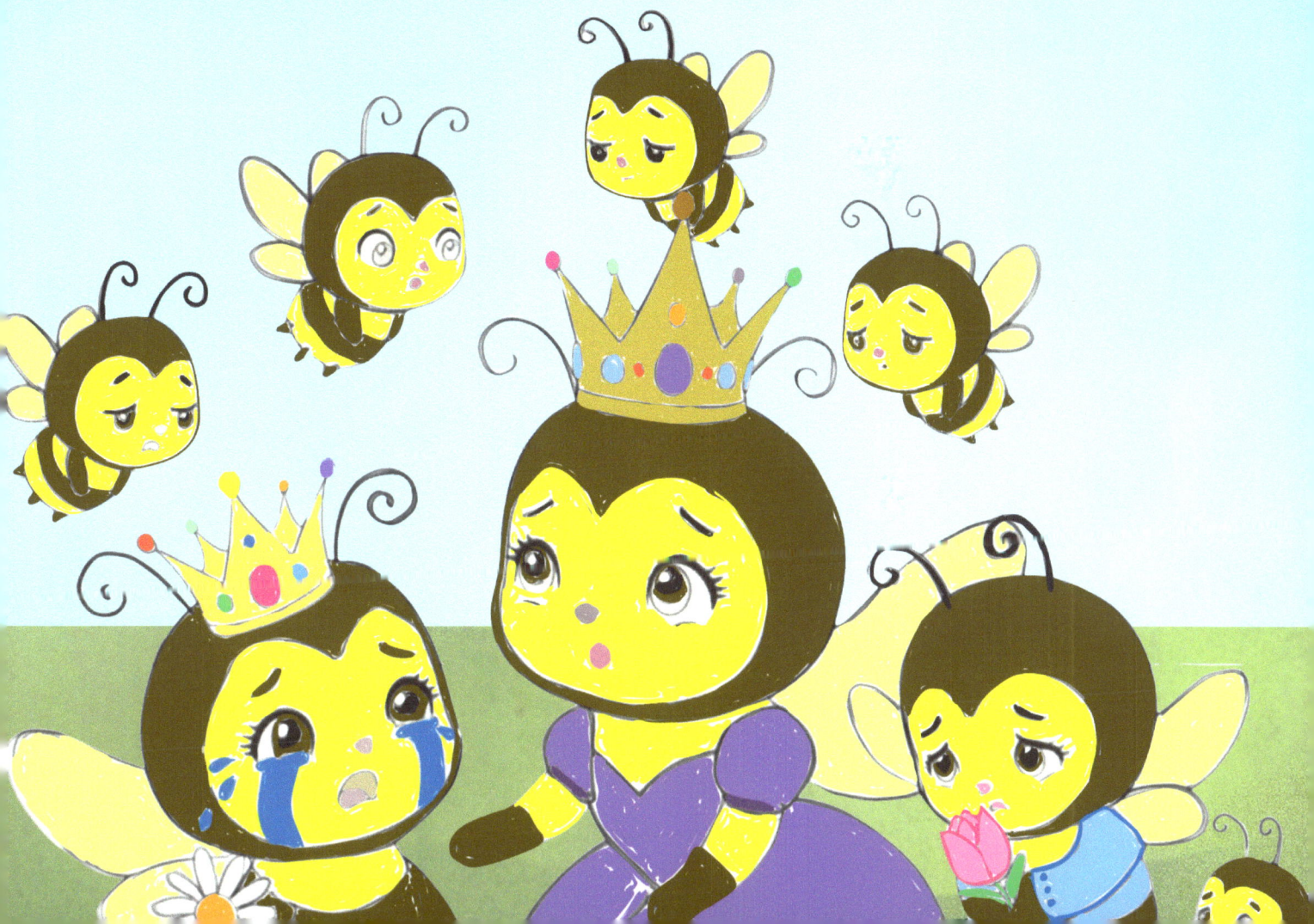

"Don't worry, StayC Bee," said the worker bees. "You'll be okay!" But StayC Bee was frightened. With Queen Bee and Sir Scot by her side, she went to the Royal Bee Hospital.

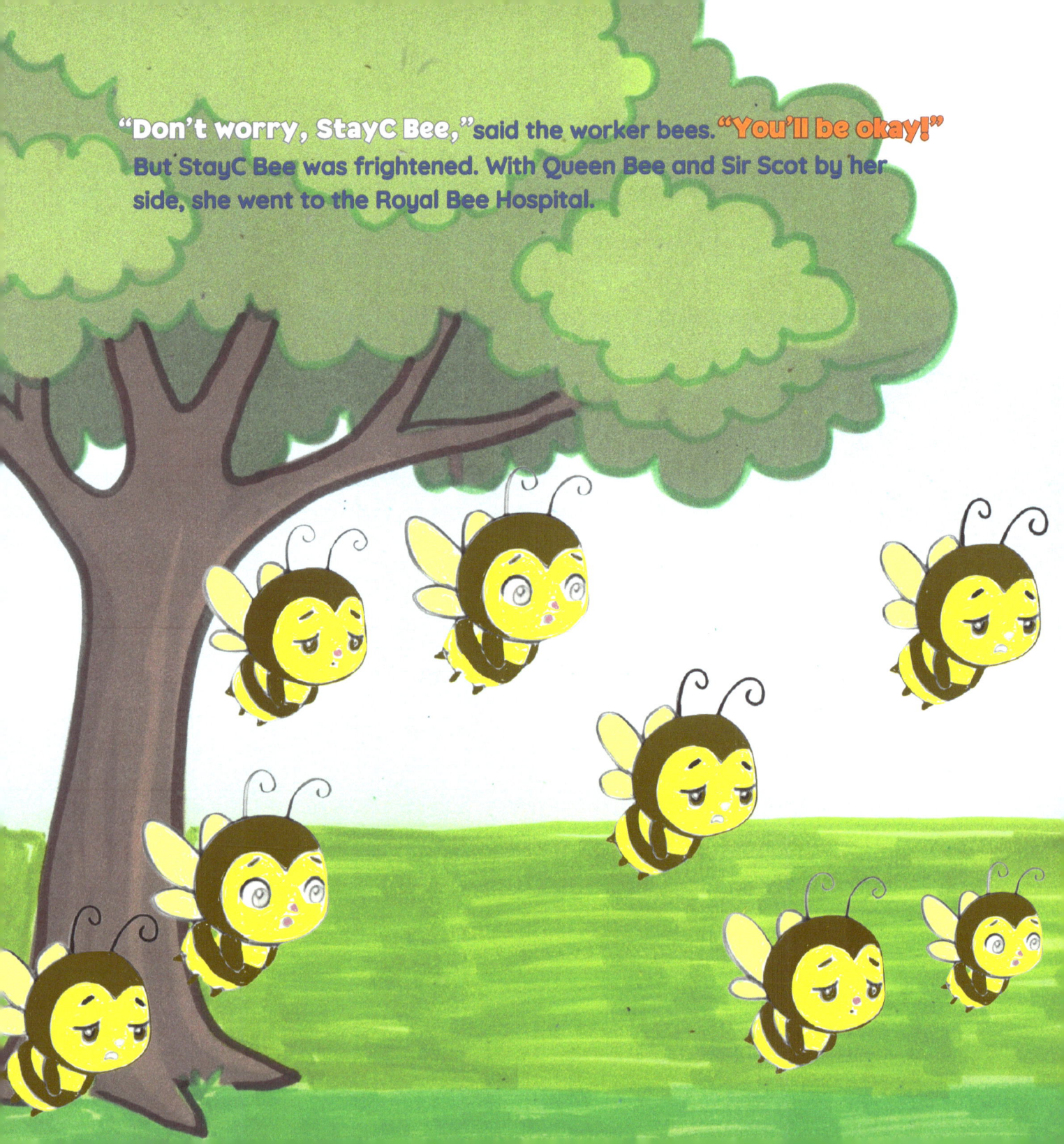

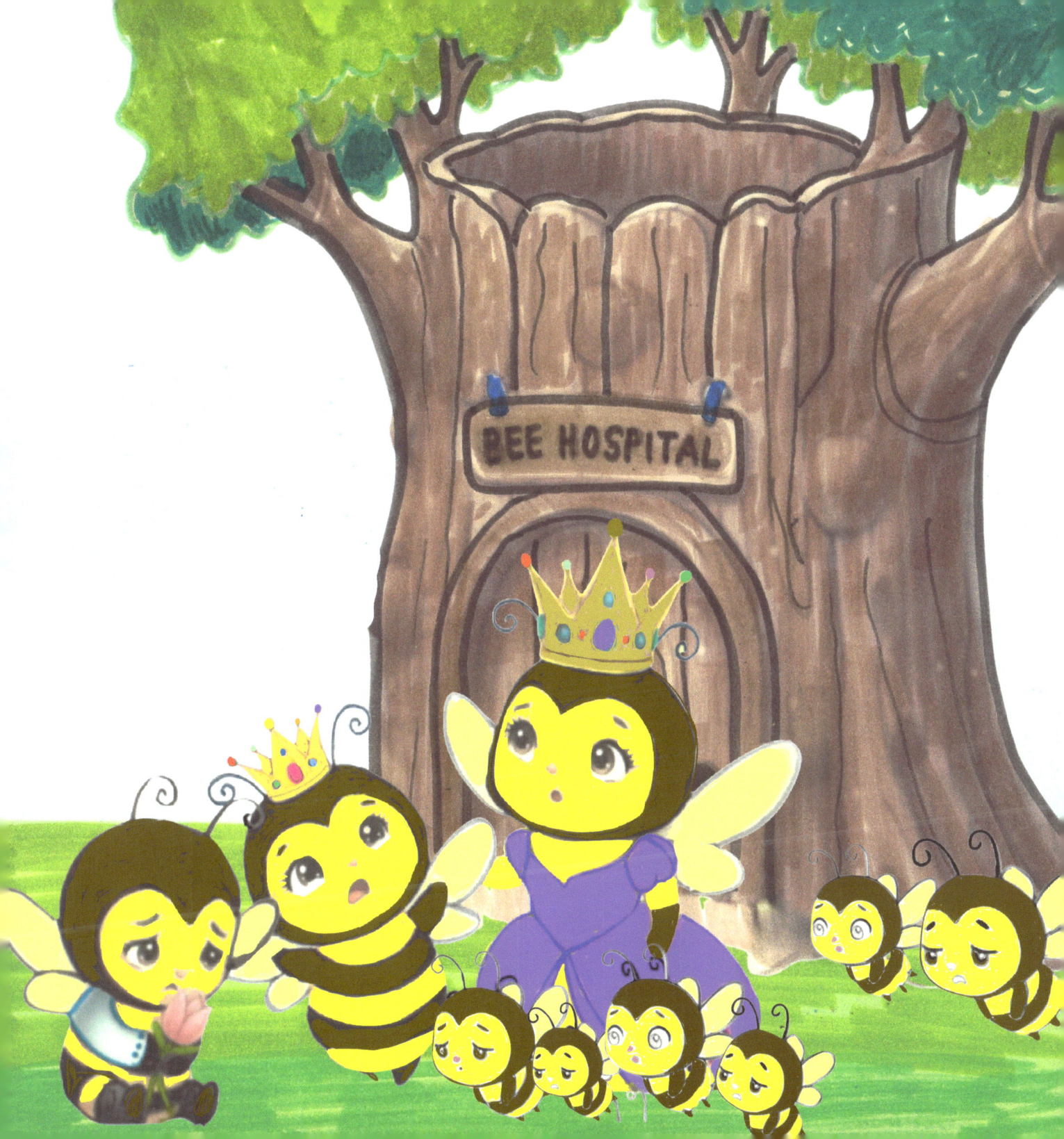

The doctor bees were gentle and kind. They ran some tests and soon discovered that StayC Bee had something called cancer. It was a sickness that would take time and medicine to heal.

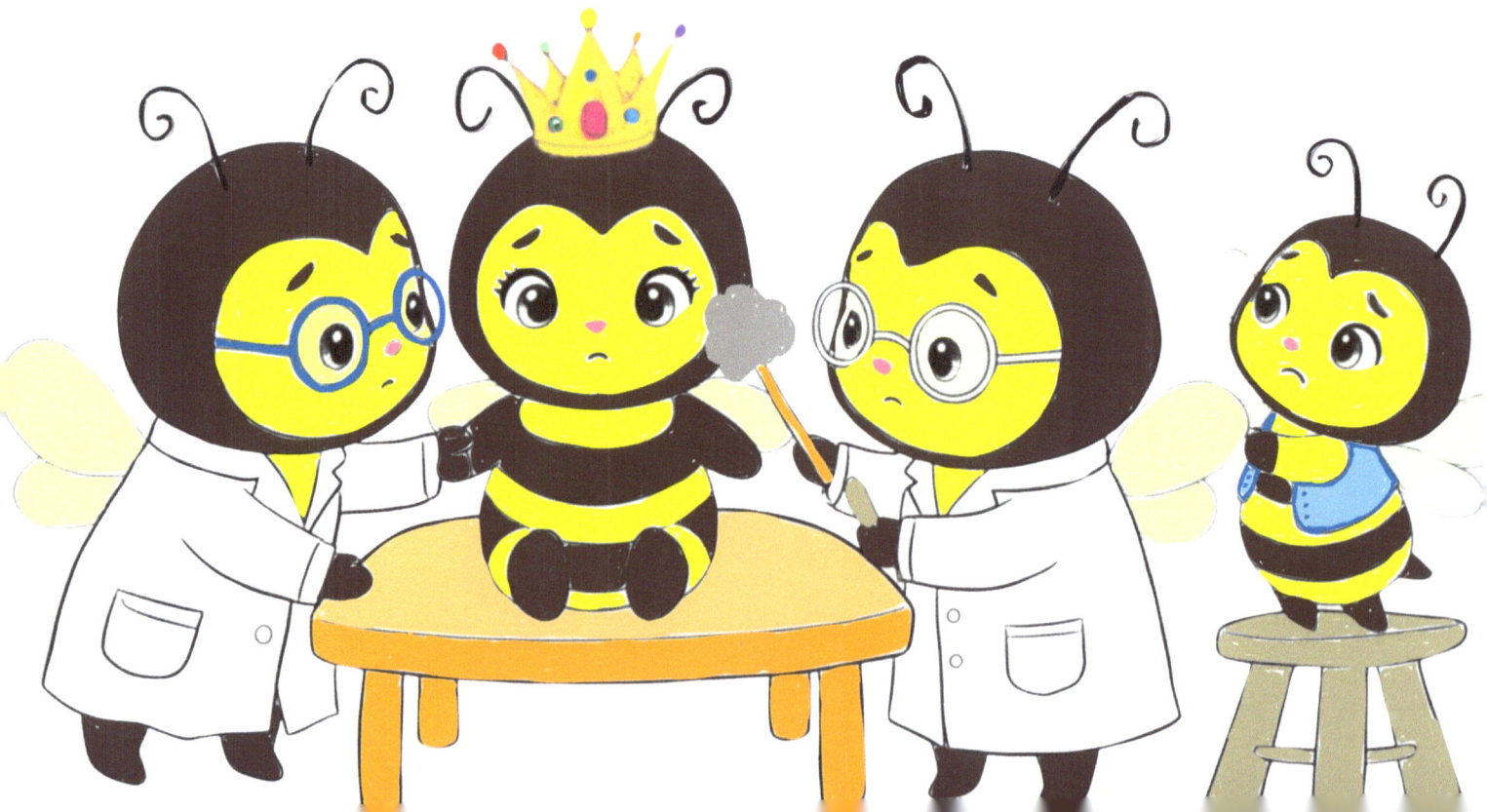

The doctor bees gave her a special medicine. It was a thick, dark honey. It didn't taste very good, and sometimes it made her feel tired and sick. They also told her that she might lose some of her pretty, soft fuzz.

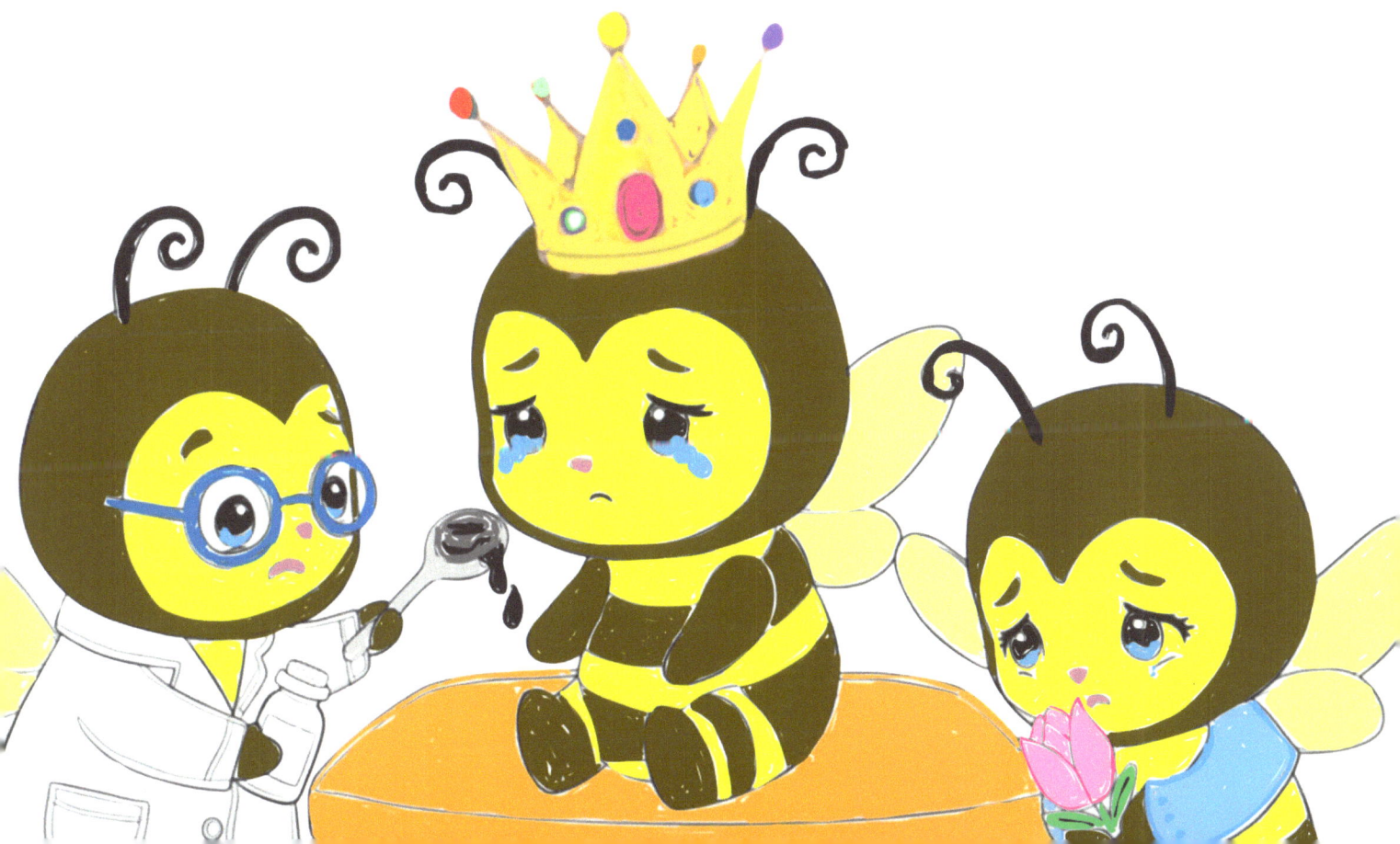

At first, StayC Bee felt scared. What would happen to her garden while she rested? Who would make sure the flowers got their morning songs?

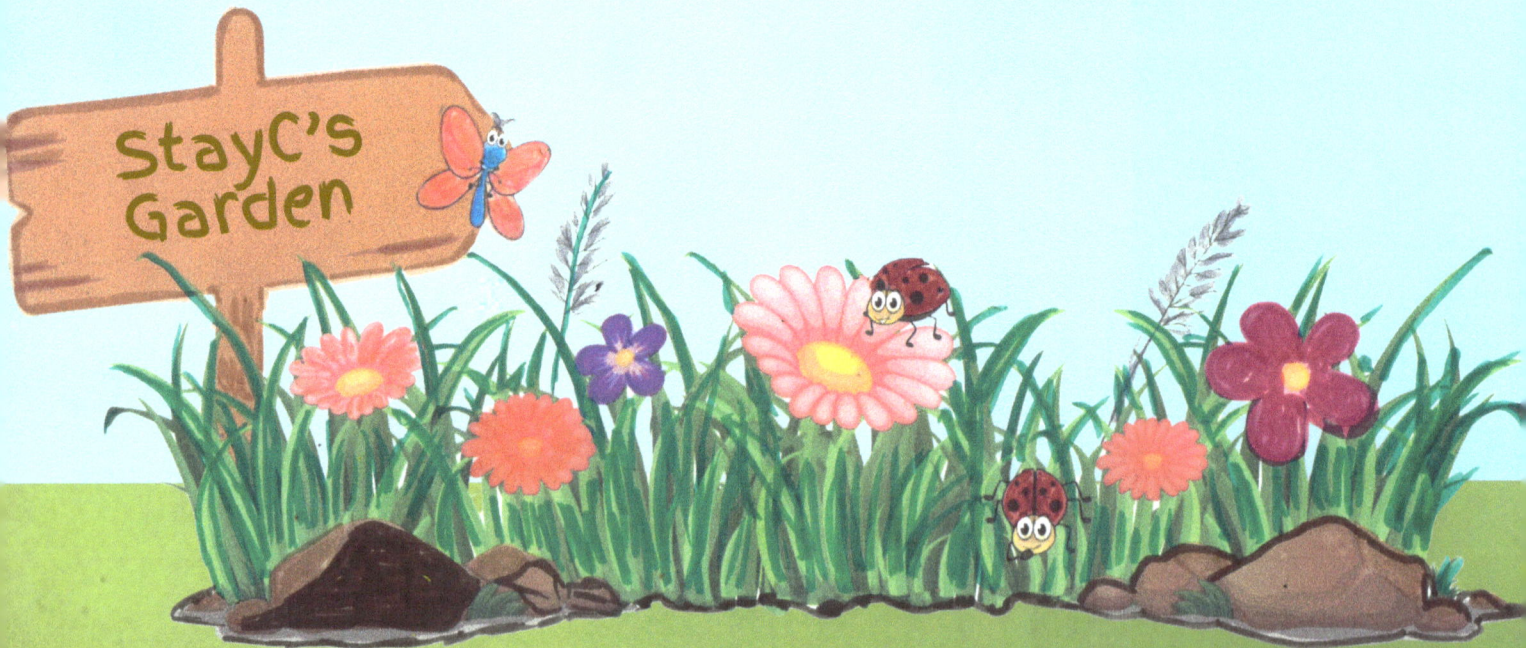

StayC's Garden

But Sir Scot promised, "Don't you worry, StayC Bee. We'll take care of everything. You just focus on getting better." He kept his promise. Every day, he and the worker bees tended to the garden, singing StayC Bee's favorite songs to every flower.

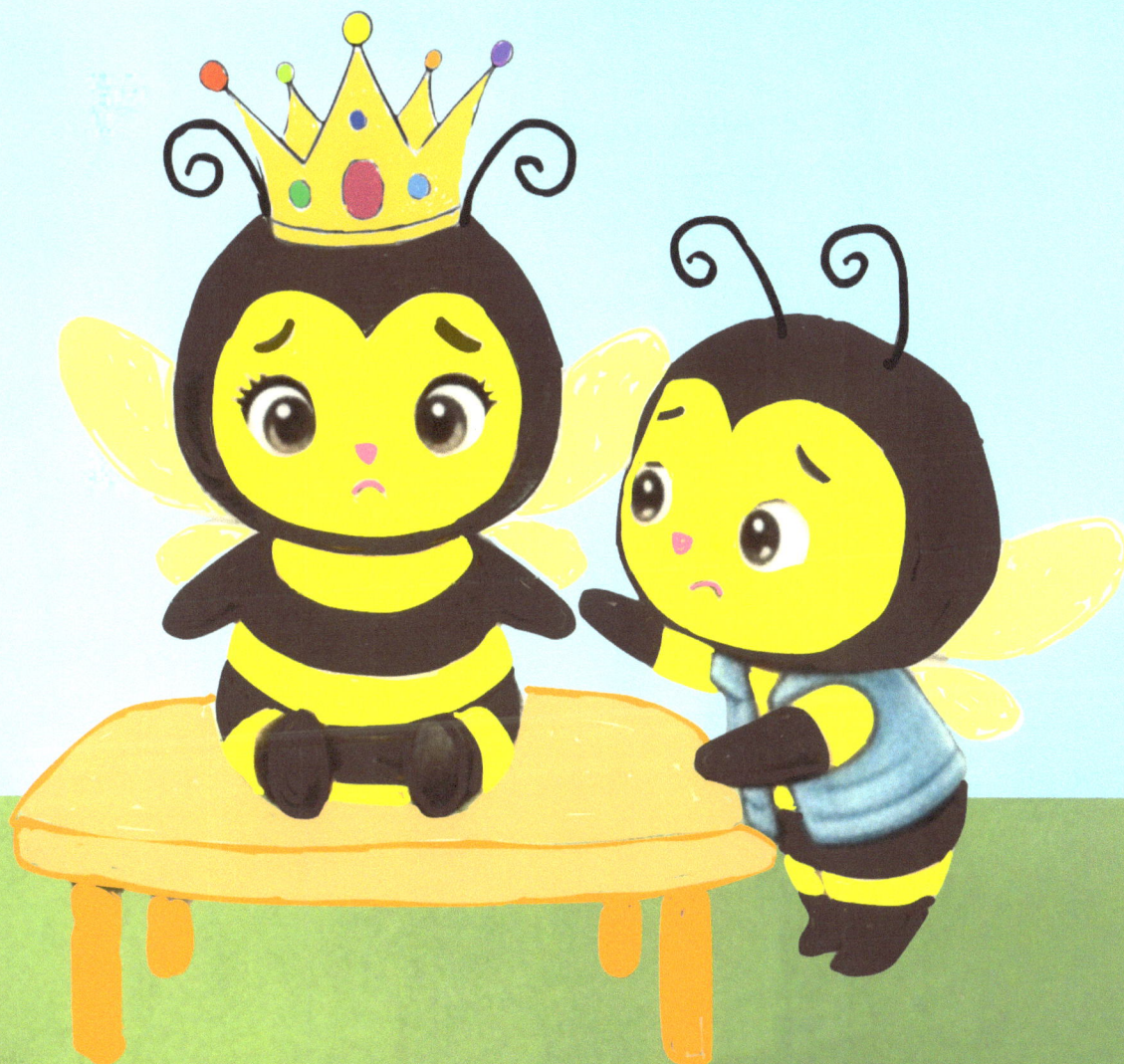

After gardening, they went to visit her. They told funny stories, sang songs, and watched StayC Bee's favorite "FishTV," a beautiful tank of colorful fish that sparkled like jewels.

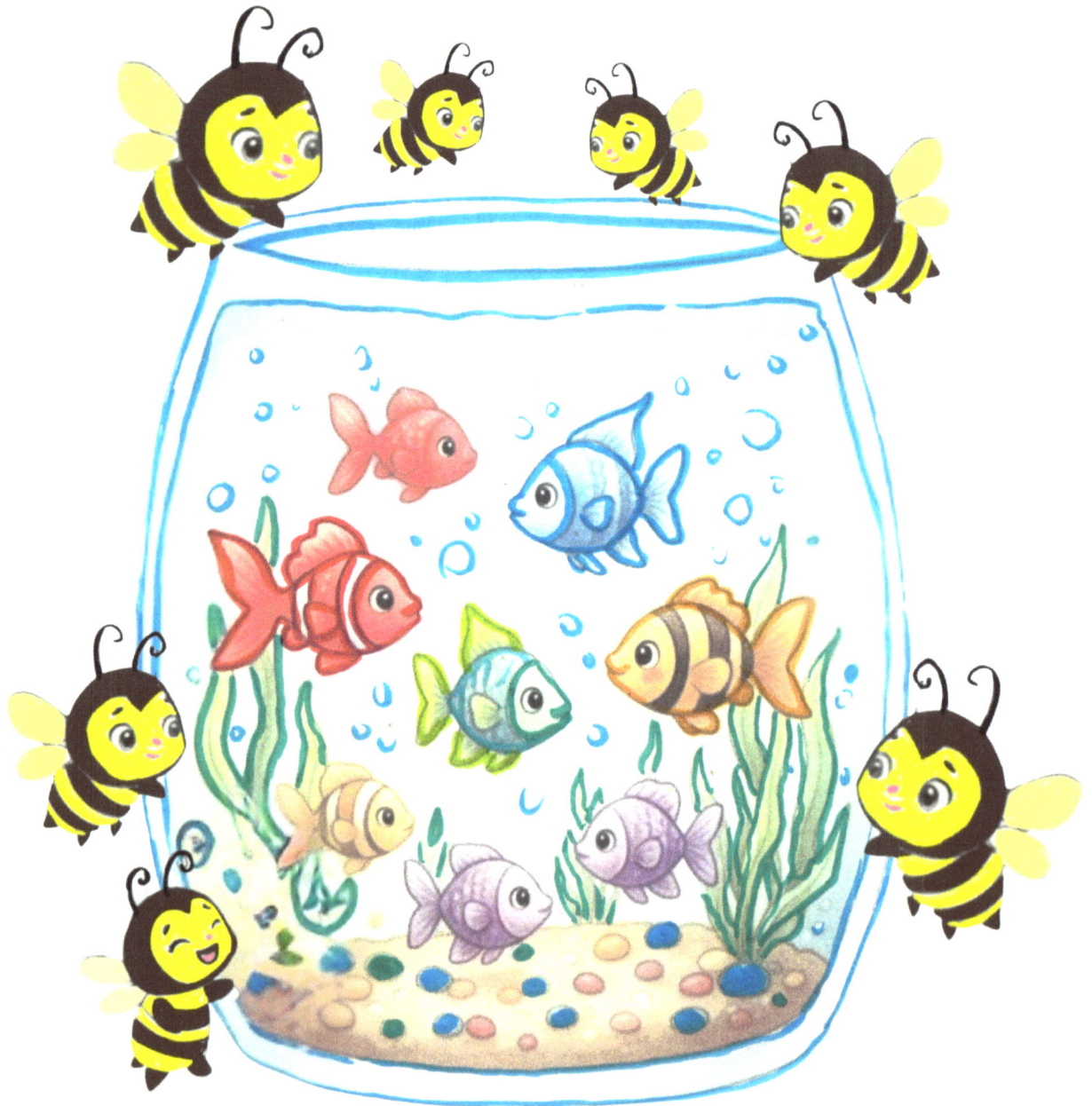

Even on the hard days, StayC Bee never stopped smiling. The love from her mom and her friends filled her heart with sunshine, even when her wings felt heavy.

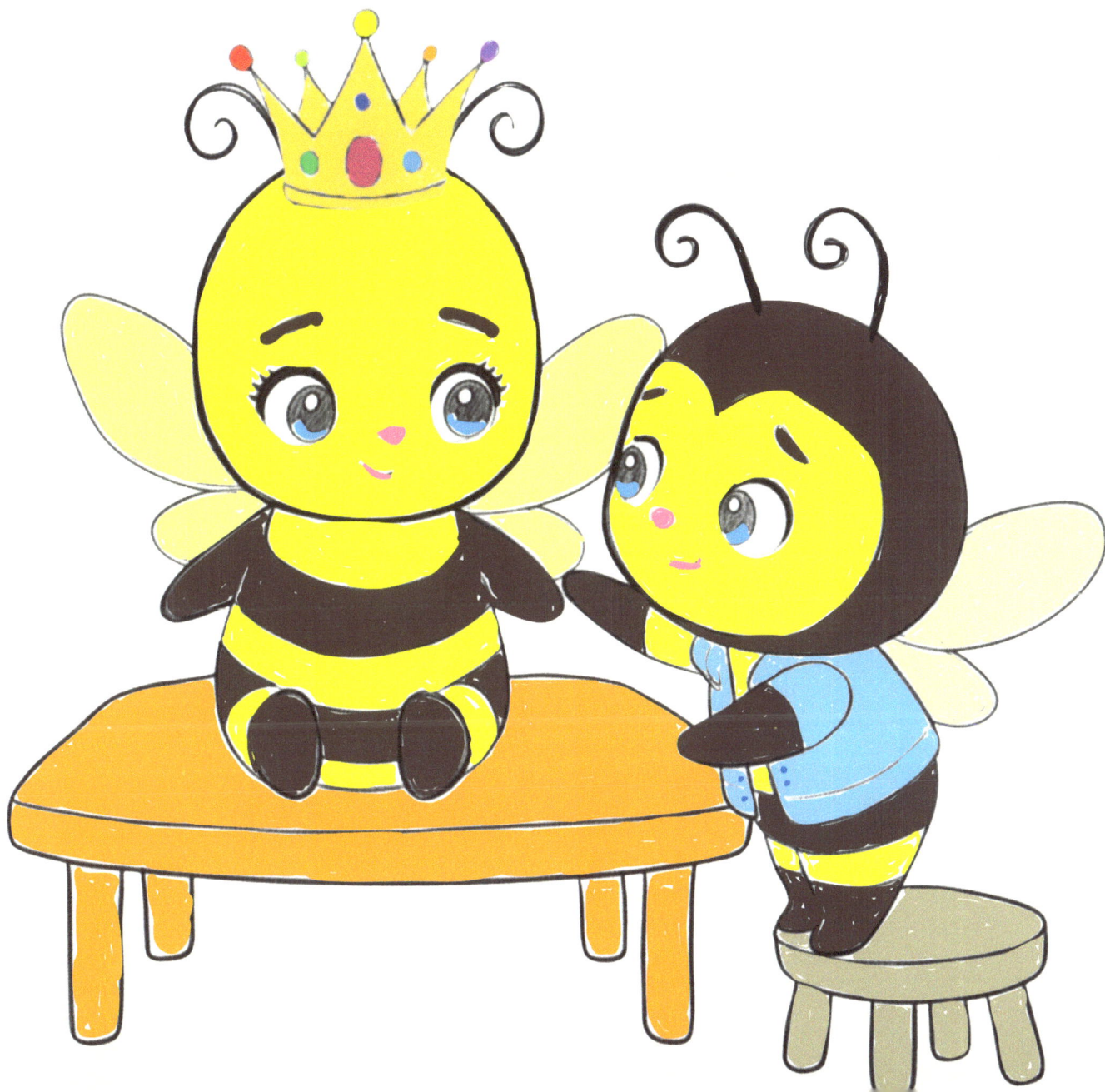

Little by little, the yucky medicine began to work. The sick cells went away, and one bright morning, StayC Bee got to do something very special. She rang the **Golden Cancer Bell!**

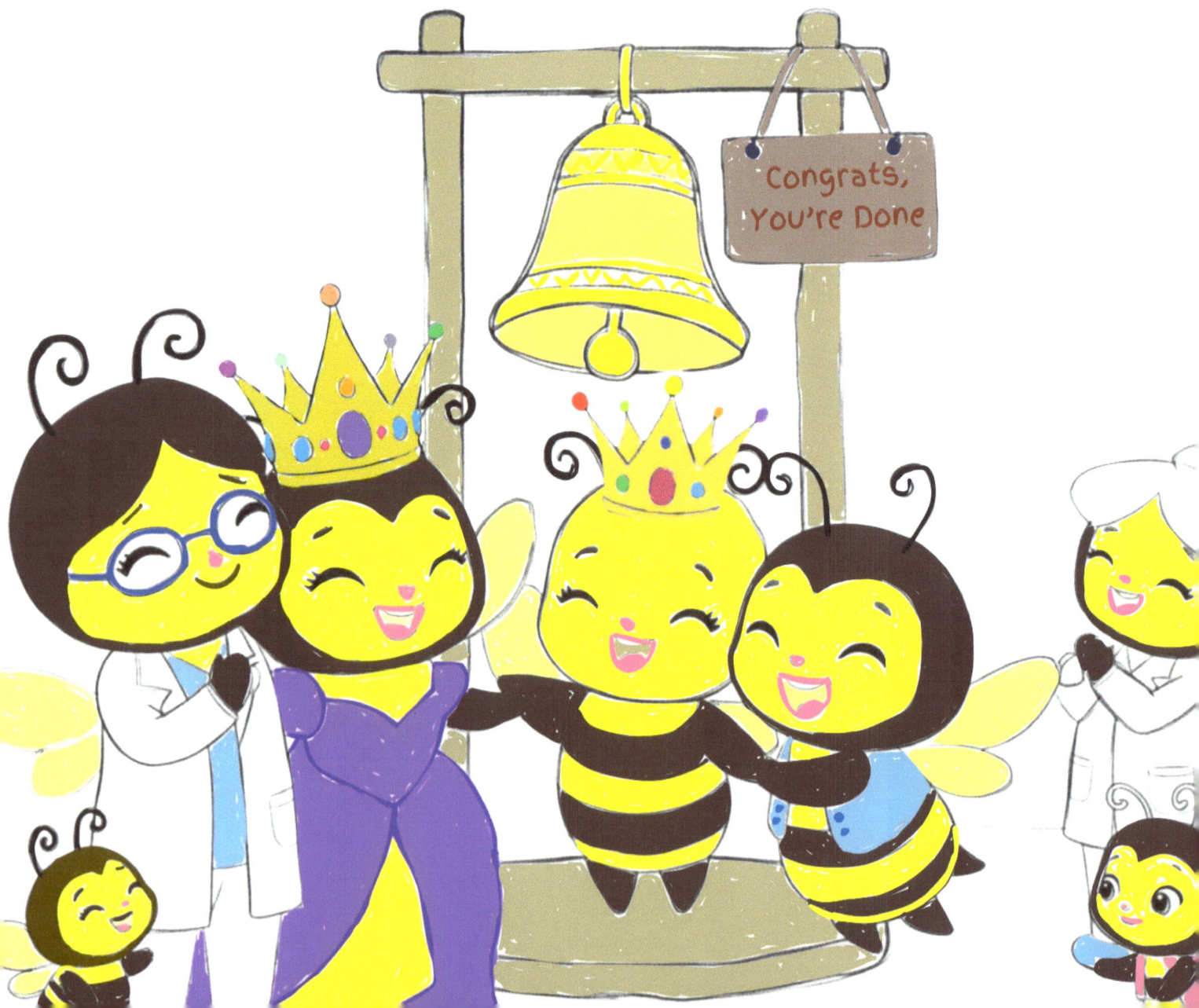

Congrats, You're Done

Ding! Ding! Ding!
All the bees in the hospital cheered.

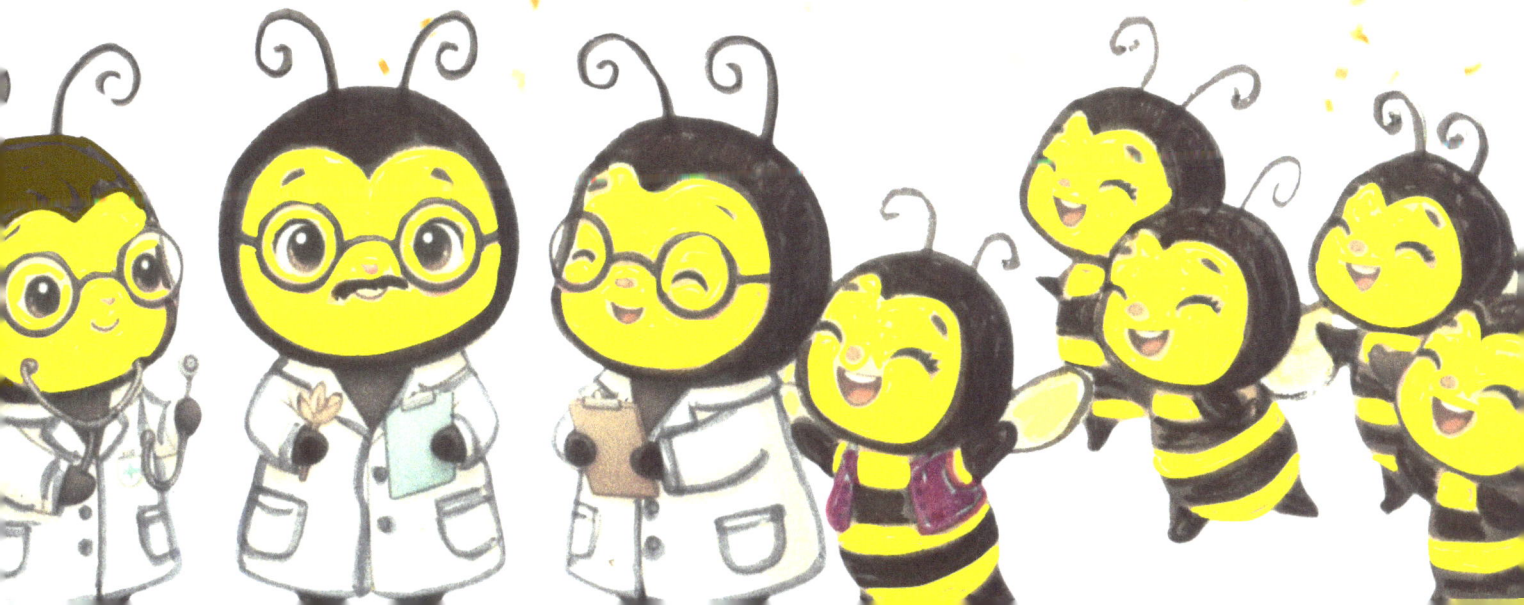

When StayC Bee and Sir Scot flew home, the whole garden was glowing with fireflies and lanterns. The hive was decorated with golden petals and ribbons. Every bee buzzed with joy!

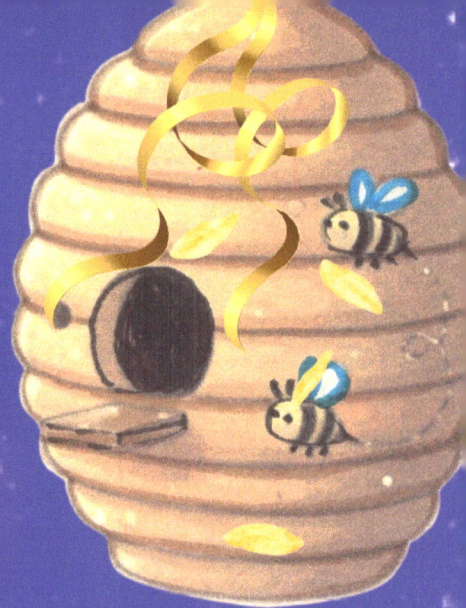

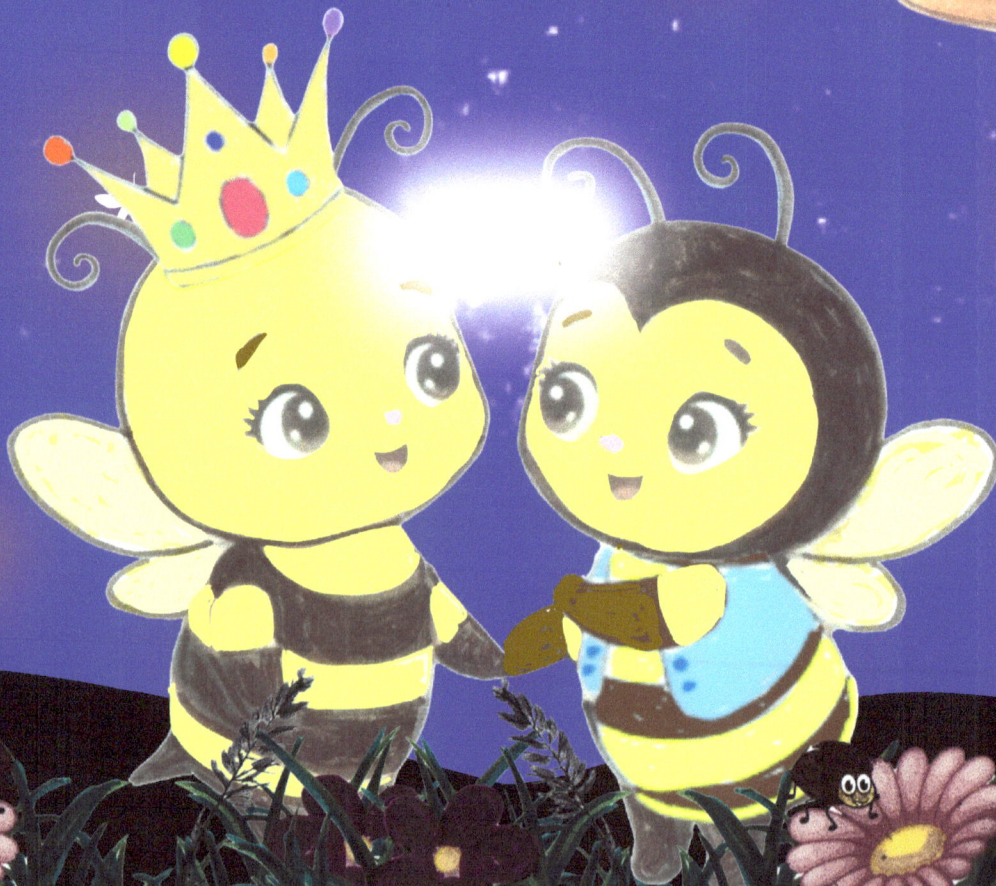

Soon, Queen Bee threw a big party for StayC Bee. Everyone in the hive was invited. StayC Bee, wearing her sparkly golden crown, looked at her friends and said softly, "I learned that being brave doesn't mean you're never scared. It means you keep going with love, hope, and a little help from your friends."

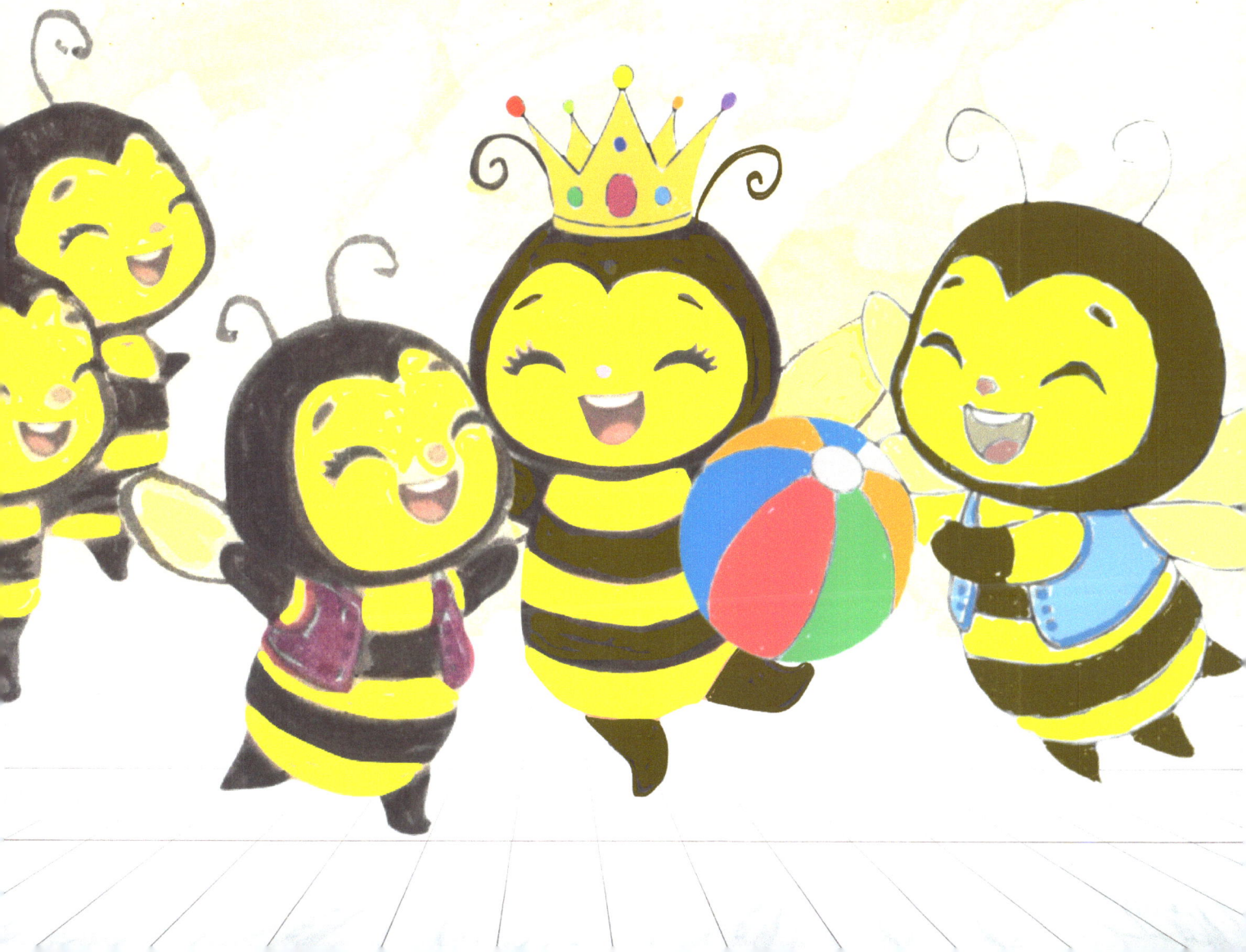

The hive buzzed happily once more, and the garden shimmered under the moonlight.

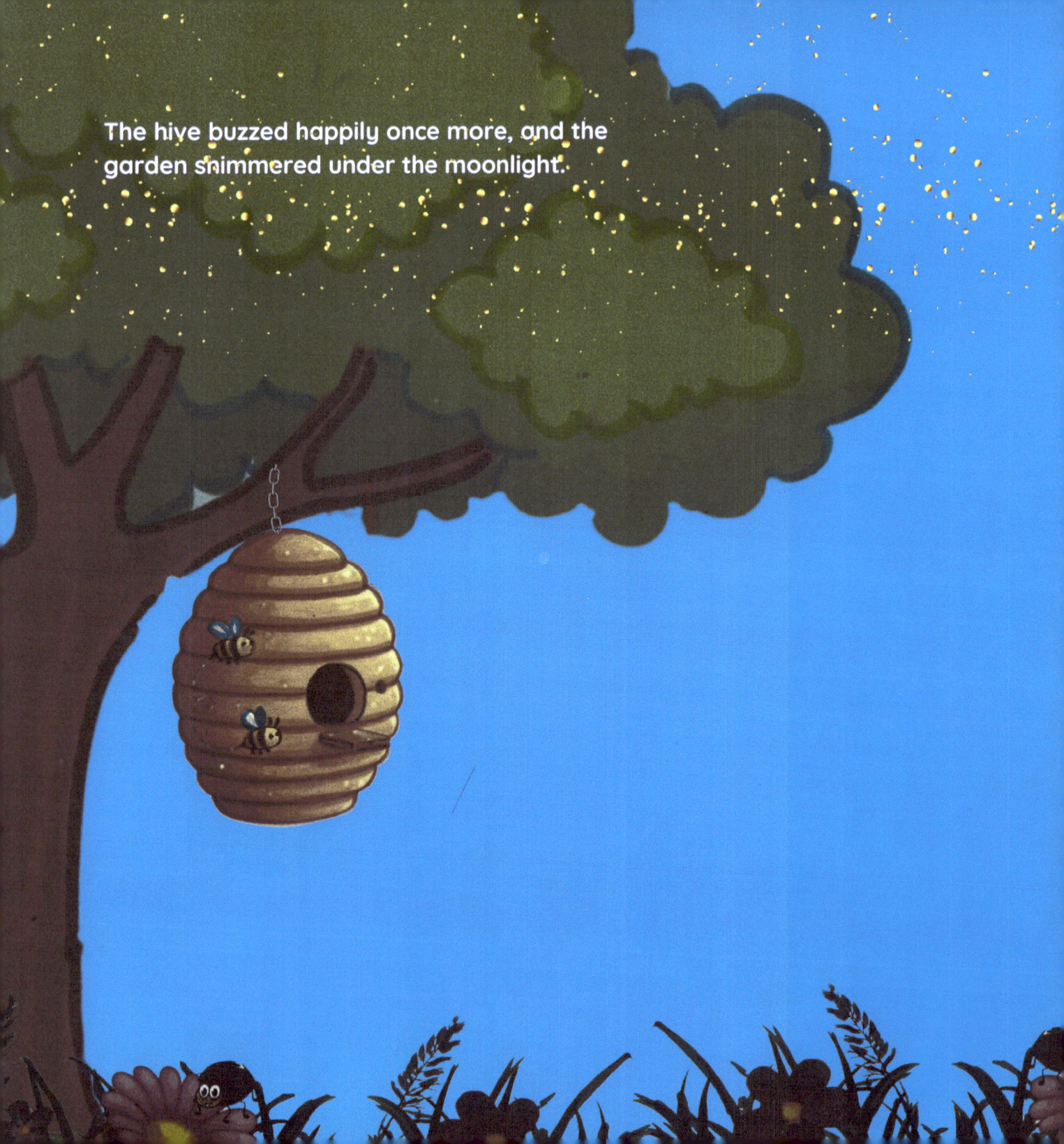

StayC Bee and Sir Scot smiled at each other. They knew that together, there was nothing they couldn't face.

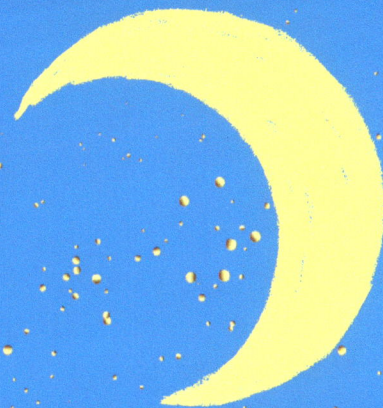

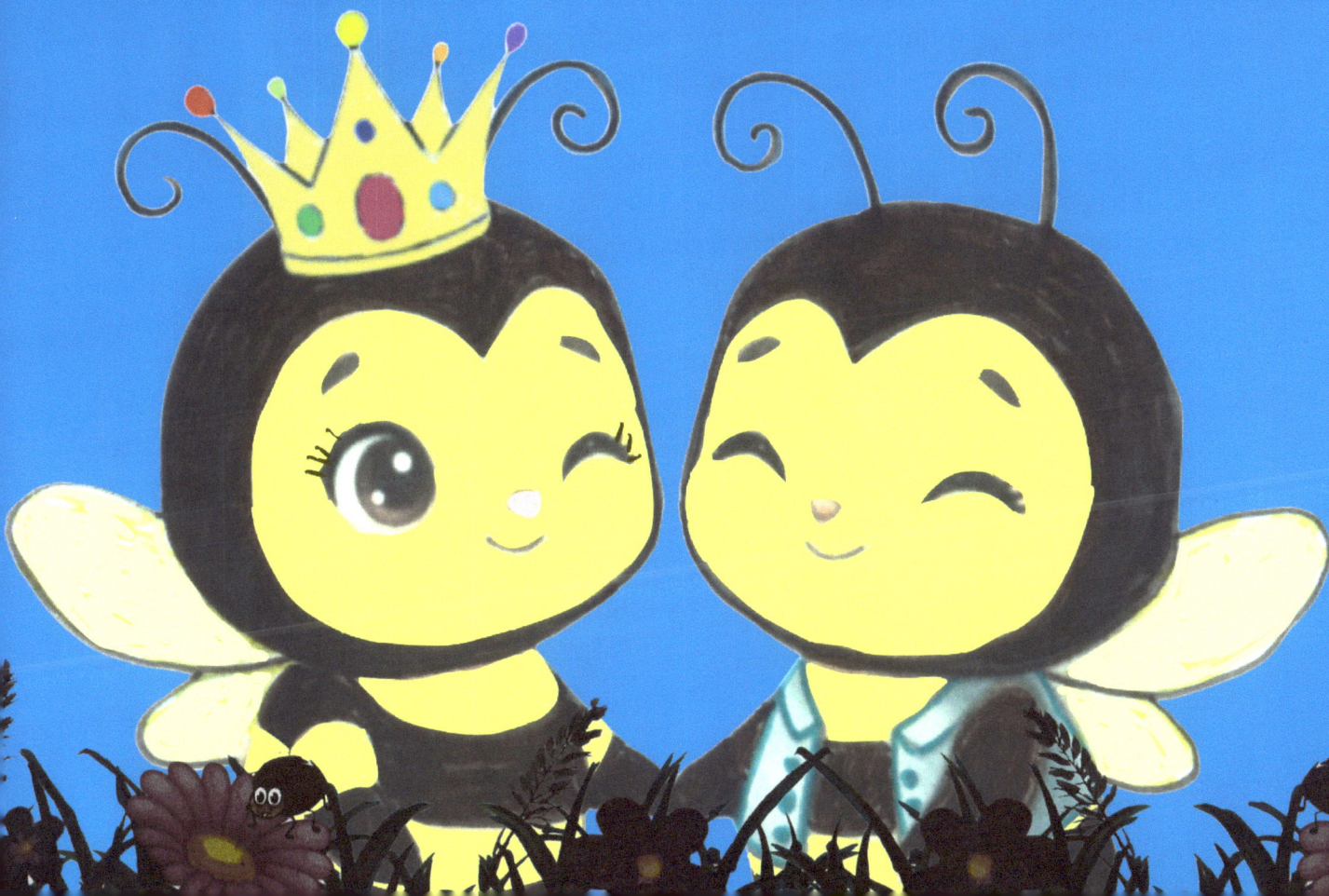

About the Author

Stayc Sharrow is a four-time cancer survivor living with heart failure caused by her treatments. First diagnosed with stage 4 Hodgkin's Disease and given eight weeks to live, she defied the odds through an experimental FDA treatment and was cancer-free a year later. Over the years, she has overcome three additional cancers and became the first woman to receive cardiac stem cells to repair heart damage.

Crowned Ms. Achievement Universe 2023, Stayc has walked in New York Fashion Week and Miami Swim Week, and appeared on a Times Square billboard as a plus-size model over 50. Her platform has taken her to 42 states, where she inspires others to live courageously and fully.

As the CEO of Gymagination, a movement education program she founded in 2003, Stayc creates inclusive spaces for children of all abilities. With a background in early childhood education, behavior therapy, and as a BCBA, she integrates her personal and professional experience to champion neurodiversity.

An ambassador for Blood Cancer United, American Cancer Society, and American Heart Association, Stayc's advocacy has been featured on The Today Show, Inside Edition, CNN, FOX, NBC Nightly News, and NPR. She is also a recipient of the President's Call to Service Award for contributing over 15,000 hours of community service.

Stayc lives in Miami, Florida, with her husband, Michael, and their three dachshunds, Ulric, Ninja, and Roland.

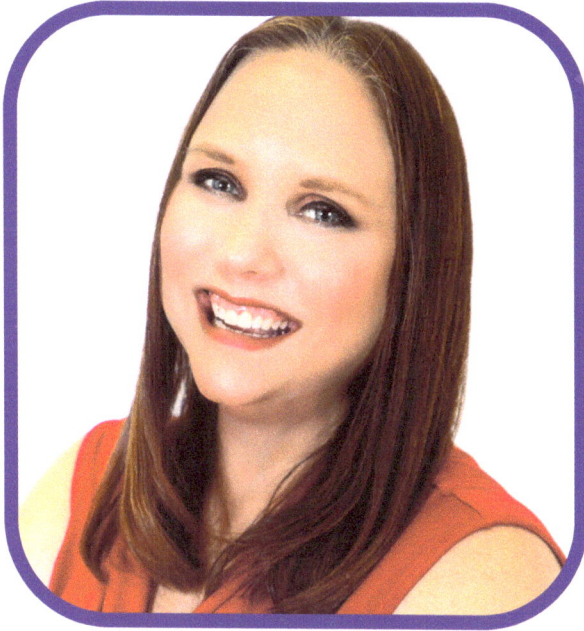
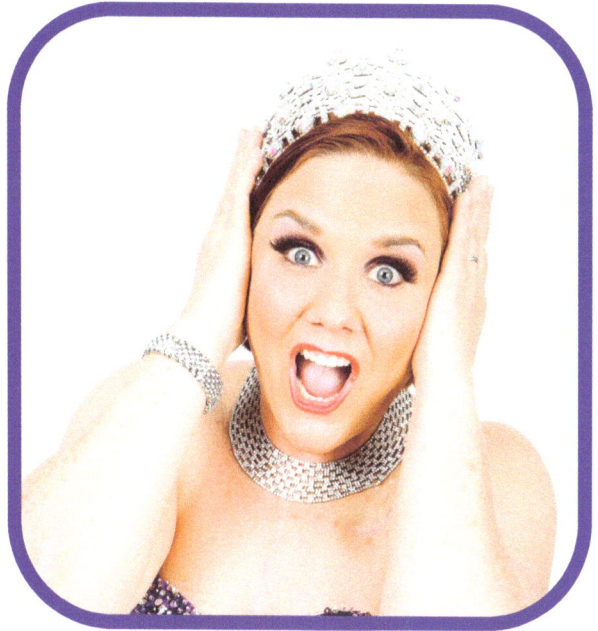

Find out more about Stayc at
queenstaycmagic.com

BELL ASTERI
PUBLISHING

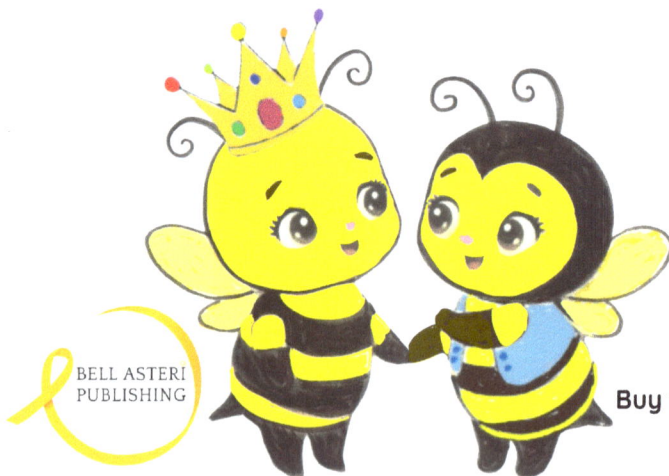

Buy the companion coloring book, "Bee Happy" at
www.bellasteri.com

www.ingramcontent.com/pod-product-compliance
Lightning Source LLC
Chambersburg PA
CBHW060856270326
41934CB00002B/158